MY FIBROID JOURNEY

Lynne Jackson

Copyright © 2019

All rights reserved. No part of this book may be used or reproduced in any manner whatsoever without the written permission of the publisher and author.

Published in the United States of America by Squinti Publishing.
www.SquintiBooks.com

(Paperback) ISBN-978-1-947350-04-5

CONTENTS

1 A HEAVY PERIOD 1

2 MY PERIODS WORSEN 4

3 MY FIRST GYNECOLOGIST APPOINTMENT 6

4 THE TEST RESULTS 10

5 A SECOND OPINION 14

6 THE SURGERY 16

7 RECOVERY FROM SURGERY 20

8 HOW THE STORY ENDS 23

1 A HEAVY PERIOD

Nina and I chatted over a goodbye coffee on that memorable morning. It was her last week with our company. She had found a better position with better pay and benefits at another firm. It was even closer to her house. I knew I would miss her terribly. She always had the juiciest gossip. Still, I was happy for her.

My period had started that morning. My flows were usually so dainty and light. I was wearing the teeniest tampon that Tampax made. As we talked, however, I could feel the blood flowing heavier than usual. Every time I laughed, I felt the blood gush out. This had never ever happened before. If I had been alone, I would have rushed to the bathroom to make sure all was well. But I was saying goodbye to my friend so I endured.

When we got up, I glanced back at where I'd been sitting. To my horror, there was blood on the plastic sofa cushion. I shrieked before I could stop myself. Nina quickly realized what was happening. She sat me back down and went to the restroom to grab paper towels. She helped me clean up the seat. I will be eternally grateful to her for taking everything in stride and not making me feel even more embarrassed. She told me the same thing had happened to her.

Fortunately, I was wearing black pants so the stain didn't show. I made my way to the restroom and cleaned up. I went to my office in the next building and grabbed my purse which had extra tampons in it. They were all designed for light flow so I knew it was a temporary solution. I left work and went to the nearest Walgreens. I bought super tampons and pads and went back to work. I skipped lunch and went home early.

Thus began a period of two years where I bled every twenty four days like a stuck pig. I bought the ultra pads and the heaviest tampons. Still, there would be four hour stretches where I had to sit on the toilet because the volume of blood going out was too much for the biggest tampon and pads to handle. Blood clots the size of an egg would plop out into the toilet bowl. The accompanying cramping made things even worse, although this had been a constant since my teenage years.

I couldn't sleep through the night. Every few hours, I had to wake up to change tampons and pads. At some point, I even tried using the ultra pads on top of diapers, so that if I slept through the wetness, at least I wouldn't get stains on my bed.

I thought at first that this change in my periods was due to strenuous exercise. I had started doing cross-fit twice a week to become more fit. Six months into this time, my heavy periods started. I can only assume a correlation. I stopped doing cross-fit after a year in the hopes that my periods would return to normal. They did not. I tried altering my diet, cutting down on sugar and red meat, and eating more vegetables. There was no noticeable difference.

About a year after the heavy bleeding started, I started chewing ice. It was something I actively avoided doing before because it hurt my sensitive teeth. However, I couldn't stop myself. I would crush the ice with my teeth then quickly move the ice away from my teeth. The texture of crushed ice felt so good on my tongue. The trickle of cold water and ice down the back of my throat felt so incredibly good.

My heavy periods drastically changed my schedule. Afraid of embarrassment, I avoided going out during the first day of my period when the flow was heaviest. I had to take sick days so I could deal with things in the safe environment of home. I turned down invitations to events if I thought my period was around the corner. If I was traveling, I stayed in my hotel room, essentially wasting a day or two of travel time. I once had to deal with my period on a trans-Atlantic flight. In spite of frequent bathroom breaks, I bled through and stained the seat. I have never been so embarrassed.

Accompanying the heavy bleeding was a general fatigue. I would become so weak that physical exertion of any kind required a great effort. Even getting out of bed was difficult. As the months went by, the weakness grew worse. Between the pain, the weakness and the bleeding, I basically had to hibernate during my periods.

Despite all of this, I resisted visiting a gynecologist. In fact, I had never been to one before. I couldn't stomach the thought of a complete stranger poking around my nether regions.

2 MY PERIODS WORSEN

Things came to a head after 3 years. I was eating so much ice, I could have filled up on ice alone. I even ate it when I didn't want to. It felt like an out of control addiction. The weakness started to linger past my period. I started to feel light-headed constantly. The last straw was an unpleasant tingly, crawly feeling in my feet especially when I went to bed. I looked up my symptoms and realized I must be severely anemic. I theorized this must be from all the blood loss.

I was sure I knew how to fix the problem. I started to eat a lot of red meat, which is the best source of iron which is needed for hemoglobin in blood. In the space of 2 weeks, I put on 5 pounds. I realized this was not a sustainable solution. I could only eat so much meat. I forced myself to eat other foods rich in iron, even when I wasn't hungry. I put spinach in my omelettes, even though I hate my omelettes this way. If I had stomach room to snack after eating cups of ice, I would eat nuts and other iron-rich snacks. The sensation of eating for nutrition rather than enjoyment was unpleasant.

My research showed me that possible causes of heavy bleeding, or menorrhagia, include uterine fibroids, hormone imbalance, and cancer. I was still hoping it was just a phase, regardless of the cause.

We had a house guest around this time, and my period reared its ugly head. I used a menstrual cup to measure my flow. The menstrual cup websites said a normal flow was about 30 ml per period. I was averaging 15 ml every 45 minutes on the first day of my period. This helped me realize my situation was far from normal. I bled so heavily that I had to sequester myself in my room, feigning illness and avoiding my guest. This was the last straw for me. I could not live a normal life because my period was now the boss of me. I scheduled an appointment with a female ob-gyn nearby.

3 MY FIRST GYNECOLOGIST APPOINTMENT

I was nervous going in to my appointment. I felt like a virgin about to have sex for the first time. I expected things to be unpleasant and uncomfortable, maybe even embarrassing. But I needed to be normal again and this was the only way I knew to get my life back.

The nurses were professional and friendly. They told me how everything was going wrong at the office that day. Their web system was down. One of the toilets was broken but they assured me they had another working toilet. I didn't understand why all this talk of toilets. Then one of the nurses took me to the working toilet and told me where to put the sample after I was done. What sample, I asked. Apparently, I had to give a urine sample. Luckily, with all the ice I had eaten that day, I had plenty of urine in reserve. I peed and left the sample in the right place.

I met with the doctor next. She asked me to take off my underwear and put my feet up in stirrups. It was my first time so in my nervous state, I disrobed completely. I'm sure she was very surprised when she returned to the room and found me completely nude.

As I explained my symptoms to her, I could see her practically rubbing her hands together with glee. As a fellow scientist, I understood her intellectual excitement. But I had lived with this condition for so long that I was over it, and I just wanted her to help me fix things. She asked me if I had been chewing ice. When I responded yes, her excitement grew even more. I was glad at least one of us was enjoying this.

Finally, she moved to examine me. She asked me if I had ever been told I have fibroids. I responded that this was my first ever visit to a gynecologist. She stopped in her tracks and asked if I was sexually active. I responded I was married, so yes. She felt my uterus through my tummy and told me my uterus was not overly swollen. I felt some pressure as she inserted a speculum into my uterus, and I felt a pinch as she completed the pap smear. She then lubed up her finger and stuck it into my vagina. She felt around and seemed to find nothing amiss. I didn't feel as bad as I had thought I would. I wasn't even embarrassed. Except, I wondered why I had waited so long to get help.

She told me the path forward: I was to get blood drawn, an ultrasound, then a biopsy. The results from all 3, and the pap smear and urine analysis, would give us a better idea of the cause of my problems. No wonder she was gleeful. I envisioned these tests alone costing a fortune. Except I could not put a price on my health.

I had blood drawn next. I exited happily after that. I felt so hopeful that a solution for my problems was around the corner. I returned the next day for the ultrasound. I had expected an ultrasound on the outside of my body, like pregnant women get. To my surprise, the nurse asked me to remove my underwear and put my feet in the stirrups. This time, I knew to keep the rest of my clothes on. She asked me if I had ever been told I had fibroids. I responded that I had never been to the gynecologist until that week. She stopped cold, and asked me if I was sexually active. I responded yes and asked why she was asking. Apparently they do not insert instruments into women who are not sexually active. I mulled on that while she lubed up the ultrasound equipment. She inserted the device into my cervix and took images of my uterus and ovaries from multiple angles. I looked closely at the images but they looked nothing like what I knew from textbooks.

The biopsy was the last step. The results would show whether I had cancer or not. The doctor warned me that I would likely experience cramping after the biopsy. She recommended I bring pain medication.

I was nervous on the day of the biopsy. I took my panties off and spread my legs as requested. The doctor inserted a speculum and expanded it. I felt the weird and uncomfortable pressure that comes with the speculum expansion. The nurse told me she had had the procedure before and she hardly felt anything, although others found it very painful. She warned I might bleed and pointed out a sanitary pad I could use after the procedure, if necessary.

I took a deep breath and braced myself. The doctor jabbed me with something and I felt the worst pain I have ever felt in my life. I screamed loudly. One more, the doctor told me. The second prick was just as painful. I screamed even louder. They removed the speculum and soothed me. I asked to see the specimen. It looked like a tiny piece of tissue in about 20 ml of blood. The doctor told me she was pleased with the specimen. I was pleased for her. The nurse told me to take as long as I needed.

I felt so violated. I lay on the examining table and cried my eyes out for a full minute. I hated the pain, the frustration, and the feeling of vulnerability. For the first time in my life, I hated being a woman. It felt like my uterus was a separate being I needed to protect.

I was worried about bleeding out on the table so I picked myself up and cleaned myself off. Sure enough, I was bleeding quite a lot and had to put on the sanitary pad. I envied those women who felt no pain and who bled little or not at all after a biopsy. On the way home, I stopped for kolaches as a treat for myself. When I got home, I cried some more. Afterwards, I ate my kolaches, then stayed in bed, too weak, angry, frustrated, and in pain to do anything besides watch tv. Once, I turned too quickly, and I felt a sharp pain in my womb where the tissue had been removed. After that, I tried to stay as still as possible. I was cramping as well but it did not compare to the pain of my period cramps. I bled for a whole day, although the pain subsided after a few hours.

4 THE TEST RESULTS

A week later, I met with the doctor and got the results of all the tests. I had fibroids: two in the walls of my uterus, one growing on the outside, and a fourth growing on the inside of the uterus. Fortunately for me, the biopsy showed they were non-cancerous. When the doctor showed me pictures of uterine fibroids, I couldn't believe my eyes. The term "fibroid" always invoked for me an image of a tiny filament-like structure. Going by the pictures she was showing me, fibroids should simply be called tumors. They are ugly masses of muscle and connective tissue interspersed with blood vessels that nourish them. They can grow very big, up to 10 pounds or more. I had suspected for a couple years that I had fibroids. If I had known what fibroids looked like, I would have seen a gynecologist much earlier.

In addition, my hemoglobin count was low. Instead of the normal 13.5, mine was at 8, which explained why I was eating so much ice. The doctor prescribed iron pills to correct that. She gave me a months supply for free and gave me a prescription for more. The pharmacy actually called me because the pills cost $400. I told them I would not be picking them up. I knew there are over-the-counter iron pills that cost much less. Of course, I would speak with the doctor first.

The doctor presented me with options for treating the fibroids. I could, of course, do nothing. The heavy bleeding and anemia would likely continue and possibly get worse. The blood vessels feeding the fibroids could be injected with blocking agents, leading to the "death" of the fibroids. The fibroids in the uterine walls would be absorbed into the body when they died, as would the one outside the uterus. However, I would have to give birth to the one growing on the inside. I shuddered at the thought. Another disadvantage was that the procedure would not prevent new fibroids from growing.

I could get a myomectomy, where the fibroids would be removed. For a woman wanting to preserve her fertility, myomectomy was the best option. I would still be able to have children, although I did not want any. However, the doctor shared her own experience where a decade after her myomectomy, the fibroids returned in full force. A myomectomy can miss fibroids that are too small to be detected. Also, new fibroids could blossom in my womb, requiring a repeat myomectomy.

Another option was a hysterectomy, where the uterus would be removed. The ovaries could remain in place. However, the ultrasound had shown a cyst on one of my ovaries. If the cyst persisted, I would have to have one or both ovaries removed. Since the ovaries are responsible for producing estrogen, progesterone, and testosterone, losing them would bring on early menopause, and could mean hormone replacement therapy for the rest of my life.

Removal of the uterus would take care of the problem

once and for all. Recovery time for robotic surgery would be 4 weeks. If there were complications and I had to have my abdomen cut open, recovery time would be 8 weeks minimum. The doctor kindly told me to think it over and let her know my decision.

I was disappointed that my doctor did not mention uterine ablation as a possible solution. When I asked about ablation, she told me they were less successful than the other methods. She really pushed hysterectomy as the best solution. I had to ask for recovery times for the different surgeries. When I asked if fibroids were genetic, the doctor indicated no. I was surprised as my research suggested the opposite.

Once again, I sobbed all the way home. I was terrified of getting surgery especially after the pain of the biopsy. I hadn't been admitted to hospital since I was 8 years old. I never fell ill. How could this be happening? I had always taken such good care of myself. I never drank or smoked or even ate fast food. In the end, it didn't even matter. It occurred to me that the human body, while complex, is far from perfect. What was the point of fibroids anyway? I felt like I would be incomplete without my uterus. My body would be marred. I would be changed somehow. It was difficult to explain even to myself.

After hours of crying, yes, hours, I finally started looking at the bright side. No more periods, for life! I could wear white every day with no fear of a sudden unexpected gush of blood shaming me. I could travel without filling half my suitcase with the bulky sanitary products I needed to manage my very heavy periods. I could go swimming any time. I would no longer need to plan vacations, important meetings, brunches, etc. around my period. I could not even imagine that level of freedom. There would be no more cramps, no more destroying my liver with pain pills every 21 days. No more days spent in hibernation as I dealt with pain and blood gushes in private. I knew that a hysterectomy would be my choice. My husband was on board, not wanting any children himself. But first, I needed to get a second opinion, just in case my doctor was wrong.

A friend told me her sister had gone through something similar. In her case, she had ignored her symptoms for many years and by the time she sought help, the fibroids had grown so much that they had become one with the uterus. The doctor had no choice but to remove the uterus completely even though the patient had requested a myomectomy.

As I took the once-daily iron pills, my desire for ice diminished slowly. I still yearned for ice until a couple weeks had passed. But finally, I had no desire left for eating ice. Slowly, my life became my own again.

5 A SECOND OPINION

Surgery is no joke. My husband and I decided that a second opinion was warranted. I found another doctor and asked for a diagnosis. I explained about my heavy periods. She had the nurses run ultrasounds on me. This time, I had one on top of my abdomen, and one inside my uterus. They found five fibroids.

So, there was no denying it. I had fibroids, at least five of them. When I sat down with the doctor, she explained that even though they had found five, there could easily be more. She went through all the options for dealing with fibroids. She was more open than the first doctor about all the possible solutions. She talked about Lupron either by itself, or to shrink the fibroids before myomectomy. Lupron reduces the production of estrogen. She touched on uterine ablation but cautioned against it. She showed me before and after pictures. The before looked like raw steak and the after looked like cooked steak. I understood why she recommended against it. Success rates were about 85%. She cautioned against a hysterectomy as she said I was too young to have my chances of having a child completely removed.

After I told her I was against hormone therapy, she recommended a myomectomy, as that would eliminate the source of the problem. She did mention that more fibroids could grow, but I would have a few years of peace and quiet.

When the doctor explained that she would make a cut along the bikini line rather than across my abdomen, I was sold. She recommended that so that I would be able to wear swimsuits without scars showing. It sound like such a small thing but that's what convinced me that this doctor was the right choice. She cared about my health and even my feminine vanity. I scheduled the surgery for a month from then.

6 THE SURGERY

Four days before the surgery, I went to the hospital for a pre-op test. It was a struggle but I managed to get past the registration desk without paying for the surgery in advance. The nurse drew blood, and took my weight. A couple of days later, I took my husband to meet the doctor so she could explain the procedure to him as well.

Finally, the dreaded day of the surgery arrived. I won't bore you with the infuriating details of dealing with the hospital billing staff. Suffice to say, they had no idea what they were doing and I felt like I was being shaken down. After the unpleasantness, I was prepped for surgery. As instructed, I had neither eaten nor drunk anything for the previous twelve hours. I was given a pill to prevent my stomach from secreting acid for a few hours. The doctor came by and she gave me more information on the surgery. I was her third surgery of the day, and it was only 8:30 am.

The anesthesiologist came by and asked for my permission to inject my sides with nerve blocker to help with pain management. This was recommended by my doctor.

The nurse anesthesiologist came by later with forms for me to sign in case I needed a blood transfusion during the surgery. I told her,

"You do whatever you need to do to make sure I'm ok."

I signed all the forms.

The nurse asked me if I was nervous. I had been holding myself together but that unexpected question made me lose it just a little. I shed a tear or two then took a deep breath and pulled myself together.

I was so nervous although I don't know how to explain why. It was fear of not being in control, other people holding your life in their hands, fear of not waking back up, fear of complications, fear of being in pain, just a general fear of the unknown. It's an experience you have to go through to really understand. I have watched people on TV get ready for surgery but I never understood the level of dread they felt. It made me wonder how people could chose elective surgery for vanity reasons. I am honestly still traumatized from the experience. Whenever I think about it too much, or when I see people on TV about to go into surgery, I get really emotional. Facing death is humbling. I was not ready to go yet. There were so many things I wanted to do. I needed more time.

The nurse was kind. She reassured me that they would do their best to make sure I was ok. I was wearing a beanie hat. I asked her if I should take it off. She patted my head kindly and told me I could keep it on. That made me tear up some more. I can't for the life of me remember her name but I am grateful for her kindness to me.

Finally it was time. I said goodbye to my husband. I was

wheeled into the operating room. All I remember is a mask being put over my face. I don't remember what the room looked like or who was there. Next thing I remember, I was in the recovery room. I had no dreams, no memories from my time being under.

I woke up in considerable pain. My poor uterus was cramping like crazy. This is how uteruses react when they are traumatized. I felt like I needed to poop really badly. I tried to tell the nurse who was bustling around me but my mouth was so dry I couldn't bring my lips together to say "poop." So I tried to say "number 2" but I couldn't say the "b" in "number" properly. Somehow, she deciphered what I was trying to say to her and put a bed pan under me. I promptly passed out. I came to and she was putting the Delaudid push button in my hand. She told me to press it if I was in pain. I promptly pressed it and passed out again. I woke up and pressed that button about 5 times. An hour and a half later, I was taken to my hospital room where my dear husband was waiting for me.

I was transferred to the bed. I hadn't pooped but I had bled a lot. The nurse cleaned me up and then put the Delaudid button back in my hand.

My husband once had a cat. He took the cat to get neutered. He said the look I gave him was the same look his beloved cat gave him when he brought him back from the vet. I totally get where the cat was coming from, although, of course, I don't blame my husband.

I settled in to my hospital room. I was extremely weak. Thankfully, I had a catheter in so I didn't have to get up to pee. I simply didn't have the strength. I was sad when they removed it the following morning because that meant I had to watch my liquid intake. I slept a lot that first day. I was grateful to have husband there. Even though I couldn't talk much, I was glad he was there to make sure I was ok.

The doctor came by at some point to tell me about the surgery. The surgery had lasted about an hour an a half. She had removed a total of fifteen fibroids. I was floored, and so was she. Apparently, so was everyone in the operating room. We couldn't understand where they had been hiding. My stomach was flat and I couldn't feel them like some people can. The biggest one was 5 cm, or almost 2 inches, across.

The pain blockers injected into my sides worked wonders. After the first 2 hours of recovery, I never needed pain medication. I was hooked up to a Delaudid IV but I never needed the button. I was in a lot of discomfort though. Stopping digestion, even for a short time causes gas buildup in the gut. The movement of gas through the gut is extremely uncomfortable, sometimes to the point of pain when there is a sudden sharp movement of a bubble of gas. My stomach became so distended that I couldn't bend forward or lie on my sides. I could only lie on my back and I quickly came to despise hospital beds. The Delaudid made me nauseated. I almost threw up once but I felt enormous pressure in my gut when I retched. After that, I knew I couldn't afford to throw up. It felt like I would rip out my stitches. Sneezing and coughing also hurt. It felt like a cruel joke when the hospital ac gave me a tickle in my nose and I had to sneeze very carefully for a few days.

I was encouraged to walk often, starting the morning after my surgery. Walking helped move things around my gut. When I finally passed gas on the second day, I don't know who was more excited, me or my nurse. I had to take medication to soften my stool. When it finally came, that was another moment of celebration. After that, I was cleared to go home.

7 RECOVERY FROM SURGERY

After I got home, I had extra strength Motrin and oxycontin which the doctor prescribed but I didn't need them as I was in literally no pain. I would usually wake up to my uterus cramping but it quieted within a minute or two of me being awake.

At first, I was so weak that I couldn't change channels on tv without considerable effort. My husband had to help me take showers. Fortunately, my strength came back after a few days and I could walk at normal speed. It was a week or so before I could sleep through the night. I was so afraid I would roll to my side that I would wake up every hour or so. I also found my bed uncomfortably soft. I was much happier lying on the couch.

For the first couple of weeks, I couldn't bend. If I dropped something, it stayed there. I dropped the remote on my second night back home. Since I couldn't sleep, I needed the tv for entertainment. I didn't want to wake my poor husband as it was the middle of the night. I used my feet to pick up the remote, then I laid the upper part of my body on the bed. Finally, I moved my feet, still holding the remote, onto the bed. It was tricky to do without involving my abdomen muscles. Then I walked to the end of the bed and grabbed the remote victoriously. I got into bed, moved the covers around, and promptly dropped the remote again.

Recovery time was 4 to 6 weeks. I was not allowed to carry anything heavier than 2 pounds. The doctor told me not to even cook or do laundry. I'm glad she was explicit because I felt like I could do those things since I wasn't in pain. You would be surprised though, at all the things that require the use of the muscles in your abdomen. Even getting up from a lying position on the couch required special acrobatics mostly involving my arms and upper body so I wouldn't strain my abdomen and tear my stitches.

As ordered by the doctor, I continued to take iron supplements. I took a course of antibiotics to prevent infection. Gas-X came in handy in the first two weeks to move gas through my gut so I could expel it. I thought my abdomen would never return to its normal size. But week after week, it subsided and by week 6, it could almost pass for its normal size.

At my two week check up, the doctor was pleased. She said the cut was healing nicely. I didn't have anything to complain about so the visit was short. She gave me a four month course of birth control pills to be started on the first day of my next period.

Birth control pills made me hungry! That's probably why weight gain is a typical side effect. Five minutes after a full meal, I would be ravenous. Eating a second mean didn't help as I would be ravenous again after a short time. I usually ended up going to bed hungry. After the four months were over, I had put on over 15 pounds.

The Pill has another big disadvantage: it has to be taken every day at the exact same time. Missing a day or taking the Pill at the wrong time renders it less effective or even ineffective. It is so inconvenient to have to take a pill at the exact dame moment every day for the rest of your life.

8 HOW THE STORY ENDS

After four months, I went in for a checkup. My gynecologist did an ultrasound and did not see any fibroids. She asked if I wanted to continue the birth control pills and I declined. Six months later, I returned for another ultrasound. The doctor found at least four new fibroids. I was devastated. All the literature said the fibroids would probably grow back but not for another 10 years or so. In only eleven months, mine had returned and had grown large enough to be detected by ultrasound.

My doctor and I discussed me getting back on birth control. I did not want to take the pill so we discussed other options. We settled on an intra uterine device (IUD) as its effects would be localized in the uterus.

The insertion of the IUD was incredibly painful and I actually screamed through most of it. Fortunately, it lasts for 5 years but I can't imagine how painful it will be to remove. Hopefully, I can be put under anesthesia for that.

About a year after I had the IUD inserted, I had another

ultrasound done. The fibroids were the same size as before. The doctor did not see any new fibroids either. It appears that hormones are essential to control the growth of the fibroids. I wonder if I could have had the IUD inserted in the first place and avoided surgery altogether. The IUD has other advantages. I no longer have periods except for occasional spotting. It also provides constant contraception which makes spontaneous sex possible.

So this is how my story ends. I am in good health and the fibroids are in check. Whenever I share my story with friends, I am surprised to find that a lot of them are dealing with fibroids themselves or know someone who is. We as women need to be more open with each other about women's health issues. If you are dealing with fibroids, be sure to get multiple opinions so you can be aware of all your options.

Good luck to you all.

www.ingramcontent.com/pod-product-compliance
Lightning Source LLC
Chambersburg PA
CBHW070038040426
42333CB00040B/1718